Frequently Asked Questions

all about
NADH
(coenzyme 1)

GEORGE D. BIRKMAYER, MD, PhD

AVERY

a member of PENGUIN PUTNAM INC.   *New York*

Most Avery books are available at special quantity discounts for bulk purchase for sales promotions, premiums, fund-raising, and educational needs. Special books or book excerpts also can be created to fit specific needs. For details, write Putnam Special Markets, 375 Hudson Street, New York, NY 10014.

Avery
a member of
Penguin Putnam Inc.
375 Hudson Street
New York, NY 10014
www.penguinputnam.com

ISBN: 1-58333-076-3

Printed in the United States of America

10 9 8 7 6 5 4 3 2

Series cover designer: Eric Macaluso
Cover image: Jack Ribik

Contents

Introduction

If you could take a natural substance that occurs in every single cell to increase your overall energy, would you? If you could take a natural substance that boosts the immune system and protects your cells from damage, would you? If you could take a natural substance that enhances your cognitive capability and improve your memory, would you? Most people would answer, "Of course."

I'm happy to report that there is a natural biological substance that offers all of these benefits. That substance is NADH, the abbreviation for nicotinamide adenine dinucleotide with high-energy hydrogen. NADH is also known as coenzyme 1, and a growing body of scientific research and physicians' experience shows that it has a profoundly important effect to keep you healthy and energetic.

NADH works for a number of reasons. First, it

is the driving force of cellular energy production. Second, it is a very important—if not the most important—antioxidant that protects your body from free radicals and the ravages of the aging process. It also enhances the capacity of your immune system and protects your cells from damage by toxins and environmental pollution. It even increases brain functions and cognitive capabilities. In addition, NADH protects the liver from alcohol damage, prevents the alcohol-induced inhibition of testosterone biosynthesis, normalizes cholesterol levels and blood pressure, inhibits the formation of free radicals in your body, and offers protection from certain toxins such as the AIDS drug AZT and other carcinogens without depleting the positive effects of the drug. That's quite a substance!

NADH was first discovered and identified more than ninety years ago, and it is extensively described in all biochemistry textbooks. Numerous positive effects of NADH in animal testing have been reported. It began to be used therapeutically in humans in the early 1980s.

In *All About NADH*, you'll learn everything you need to know about this amazing substance.

The first two chapters describe what NADH is, and how and why the body needs, makes, and stores energy. The following chapters provide an overview of NADH's health benefits and explain why this coenzyme does so many good things to help us lead healthy lives. Subsequent chapters cover the benefits of NADH in greater depth, especially its benefits for often disabling disorders such as chronic fatigue syndrome (CFS), depression, Parkinson's disease, and Alzheimer's disease. The final chapter tells you all about the best form of NADH to take and offers other usage recommendations for this remarkable dietary supplement. Sit back and delve into this book now, so you can understand the many ways that NADH may better your quality of life.

1.

An Overview
of NADH

NADH is a naturally occurring and very important compound found in all living cells of plants, animals, and humans. It's vital for health. This chapter will review the basics about NADH, including how and when this substance was discovered and why it is so critical for proper body function.

Q. What is NADH?

A. NADH is the abbreviation for the naturally occurring biological substance, nicotinamide adenine dinucleotide hydride. The "H" stands for high-energy hydrogen and indicates that this substance is in the most biologically active form possible. Often referred to as coenzyme 1, NADH is the body's top-ranked coenzyme, a facilitator of numerous biological reactions. NADH is necessary for cellular development and energy production: It is essential to produce energy from food and is the principal carrier of electrons in the energy-producing process in the cells. NADH is also an important antioxidant; in fact, scientists acknowledge that NADH is the most powerful antioxidant to protect cells from damage by harmful substances. In summary, NADH is a highly powerful form of vitamin B_3 commonly referred to as niacin or niacinamide.

Q. When was NADH discovered?

A. NADH was discovered in 1905 and was found to be an essential co-factor or co-partner for all enzymes in the body, and therefore is commonly known as "coenzyme 1." Since its discovery, more than one thousand different physiological functions of NADH have been detected and extensively described in all biochemistry textbooks. However, NADH was viewed as so unstable—it could react to even small amounts of exposure to heat, light, or humidity—that it could not be used therapeutically. This was the reason that NADH has not been widely discussed before.

Fortunately, in the mid-1980s, researchers used modern-day technology to develop a stable, ingestible, and absorbable oral form of NADH that can improve the level of NADH in the billions of cells that make up the human body. A safe and effective form of NADH can now be used therapeutically.

Q. What is a coenzyme?

A. A coenzyme is a substance that enhances or is necessary for the action of all enzymes in the body. Coenzymes are generally much smaller molecules than enzymes themselves. Enzymes are large biological molecules that catalyze biological processes and create products in our bodies that we need for basic survival. Without a coenzyme, the majority of enzymes in the body are useless. Enzymes can be compared to production machinery in a factory that transposes one material into another one. In living cells, enzymes catalyze the breakdown and turnover of food components into smaller units, converting food into energy and water. Enzymes can perform their work only if an additional essential factor combines with the molecule itself. This factor is called a coenzyme. Without a complementary coenzyme, enzymes will not work and, therefore, they cannot produce complete protein systems for the human body. Hence, a coenzyme is essential for an enzyme to become active. Unlike DHEA and melatonin, NADH is *not* a hormone, but a *coenzyme*.

Q. Why is NADH important?

A. NADH is biologically ranked and identified as coenzyme 1, the coenzyme or cofactor needed for numerous enzymes that are involved in the cellular energy production. A deficiency of NADH will result in an energy deficit at the cellular level, which causes symptoms of fatigue. When the body is deficient in NADH, it is kind of like a car that has run out of gasoline. The more NADH a cell has available, the more energy it can produce. Unfortunately, the production of NADH in our bodies declines as we age, and so does the production of NADH-dependent enzymes, particularly those enzymes involved in energy production.

Q. What foods are natural sources of NADH?

A. NADH is present in all living cells of humans, animals, and plants. Hence, it is present in our daily food sources. However, animal protein sources—meat, poultry, and fish—contain the highest amount of NADH. Vegetables, fruits, and other vegetarian food have a much lower NADH content. Plants need less energy to survive and no energy for locomotion or movement, so they have less NADH. Vegetarians, therefore, receive little NADH from their diets and should consider supplementing with NADH.

Many other people also can benefit from taking NADH supplements, though, for a few key reasons. First, almost all of the NADH we take in from food is destroyed during food preparation. Second, even if our diets consisted mostly of raw meat or fish (which isn't advisable), we would only receive a minimum of NADH from these food sources. Most of the NADH in these foods would be degraded by the stomach's own digestive gastric acids that break down food into its constituent parts for absorption.

Q. Who discovered how to use NADH therapeutically?

A. The NADH story began in a roundabout way in the late 1940s and 1950s. At that time, my father, Walther Birkmayer, MD, began exploring biochemical transmitter mechanisms within the human brain. His research led to the realization that injuries to the brain actually create an imbalance between various reactor substances or neurotransmitters, resulting in a wide range of patient behaviors and symptoms.

During the 1960s, my father discovered that L-Dopa (the synthesized form of the neurotransmitter dopamine) could relieve symptoms in patients with Parkinson's disease and allow these patients to experience increased mobility with less rigidity. The L-Dopa treatment, known under the brand name Sinemet, is now the preferred drug therapy for Parkinson's disease. However, L-Dopa treatment has one big drawback: It is given in very high amounts, causing an "overloading" of the body and the brain. This leads to a dangerous side effect: the production of enormous amounts of free radicals. Free radicals are highly active molecules that react with every substance in a cell and can damage cell membranes. Medical researchers also know that L-Dopa therapy becomes less and less effective over time, with more and more resulting side effects. This damage has been observed in patients with Parkinson's disease, particularly after long-term treatment.

The drawbacks to L-Dopa treatment prompted my father and me to develop a completely new treatment approach using NADH. We began using NADH in pure form for intravenous infusion in 1985. NADH worked because it naturally stimulates the body to produce its own dopamine. NADH was so unstable, though, that it needed to be given intravenously at a clinic or hospital, so this made treatment inconvenient and time-consuming. To make NADH easier to use therapeutically for our patients and others, we sought out and eventually developed a stabilized, absorbable, form of NADH that could be taken by mouth in easy-to-swallow tablets.

Q. How long has NADH been available as a dietary supplement?

A. An exclusive stabilized, absorbable, patented tablet form of NADH has been marketed as a dietary supplement in the United States since 1995.

NADH is a very sensitive substance. It degrades rapidly under the influence of light, humidity, temperature, and other factors. For example, it is degraded by milk sugar, also known as lactose, one of the classical tablet filler agents commonly used in many drugs and nutritional supplements. It took more than five years of extensive research to develop a stabilized, oral, absorbable form of NADH that does not use this type of filling agent. This special formulation is now covered by several worldwide patents and was given the brand name ENADA. To date, hundreds of thousands of consumers have experienced many beneficial effects from this product.

2.

How Your Energy Depends on NADH

The billions of cells that form tissue and organs and ultimately the human body have an important assignment: to produce energy. If our cells slow down or decline in their energy production, the most visible result is that we are tired and can increasingly experience greater overall fatigue. This chapter explains how the body produces and stores cellular energy and how NADH is vital to these processes.

Q. How does the body produce energy?

A. Bringing hydrogen and oxygen together is one of the most efficient ways to produce energy. A rocket launched into outer space is an example of energy production. All cells in our bodies use the same principle of energy production, but they do so in a sophisticated way to conserve the energy produced. NADH is the biological form of hydrogen that reacts with the oxygen we breathe in to form energy and water. The energy-producing process in cells is achieved by a cascade of reactions, which lead to the formation of adenosine triphosphate (ATP), the energy-containing compound in cells. One molecule of NADH will form three times the amount of ATP. Therefore, NADH is an extremely efficient and effective energy producer.

Q. How does the body store energy?

A. Living cells have the capability to store energy in the form of chemical compounds. When these compounds are metabolized, energy is released and used for all cellular processes. Only a few biological substances display all the features of energy-rich compounds. The most important of these are adenosine triphosphate (ATP), creatine phosphate (CP), nicotinamide adenine dinucleotide hydride (NADH), and nicotinamide adenine dinucleotide phosphate hydride (NADPH).

Q. Is ATP the most common "energy-rich" compound in our bodies?

A. Yes, ATP serves as the most common and convenient chemical form of energy stored in every cell. It's kind of like a biological battery that stores and releases energy when the body needs it. When cellular energy is required, ATP is broken down under the action of water to release energy for other processes. As already mentioned, NADH is a very efficient producer of ATP.

Q. Is NADH also an "energy-rich" compound?

A. Yes, energy is stored in the NADH molecule. When NADH reacts with the oxygen present in every cell, energy is produced in the form of ATP. One NADH molecule leads to the formation of three ATP molecules. In other words, NADH has triple the energy capacity of ATP. Furthermore, NADH creates additional energy when it reacts with oxygen and water forming nicotinamide (also known as vitamin B_3) and ADP (adenosine diphosphate). All this means that NADH is a super energizer.

Q. What is the Krebs cycle within our cells, and does it produce NADH or ATP?

A. The Krebs cycle is also known as the tricarboxylic acid (TCA) cycle and as the critic acid cycle. Hans Krebs worked out the details of the cycle in the 1930s. The cycle takes place in the mitochondria of the cell and consists of several highly technical steps involving the conversion of proteins, carbohydrates, and lipids as well as their metabolites—amino acids, sugars, and fatty acids. There is no energy produced in the cycle—only NADH, which then triggers energy production in the form of ATP. Actually, each "turn" of the cycle produces three molecules of NADH. If the body needs more and more energy (ATP), then the cycle begins to speed up to produce more NADH. As this process continues, the body begins to signal us through hunger so we can ingest more food for conversion. However, if we ingest too much food (calories), the body tends to store the calories as fat. In summary, the Krebs cycle within our cells is necessary to produce NADH, and NADH efficiently produces ATP energy. Whether NADH is produced internally within the cell or NADH enters the body from a dietary supplement, it will trigger cellular energy production. Therefore, with the proper dietary supplementation with NADH, the cells in the body can directly produce ATP energy without the constant activation of the Krebs cycle, which eventually signals hunger to the body.

Q. What role do free radicals play in energy production, and how are they created?

A. Free radicals interfere with cellular energy production by destroying many of the enzymes and energy-producing compartments within the cell. These energy-producing compartments are called the mitochondria, which as we learned previously are important producers of NADH, which in turn produces cellular energy ATP. Free radicals are continuously produced in minute amounts inside the cells during normal metabolism and also during normal activation of the immune system. However, the greatest amount of free radicals actually comes from outside our bodies. With our increasing environmental exposure to various agents such as radiation (x-rays, UV light), ozone, drugs, and other chemical toxins, free radicals continuously bombard and enter our bodies. These free radical molecules are very reactive molecules and usually consist of an unstable oxygen atom that is missing an electron. The atom with the missing electron wants to find a replacement electron from the closest molecule that is part of a healthy cell. With this constant bombardment of healthy cells, the free radical can eventually damage the healthy cell and/or its internal compartments until extensive cell damage occurs, which can potentially manifest later in life as major disease types.

Q. How does the body deal with these free radicals?

A. Fortunately, the body has several ways to eliminate or detoxify these free radicals. Antioxidants, in the simplest terms, are substances that prevent the chemical reaction called oxidation, which produces free radicals. Normally, the body produces natural antioxidants that help fight these free radicals by donating electrons freely and therefore helping to prevent harmful kinds of oxidation such as oxidation of cellular tissue. Other antioxidant protection is obtained from the foods we eat like fruits and vegetables or by taking nutritional supplements such as NADH, vitamins A, C, and E, and so on.

3.

How Your
Body Benefits
From NADH

The human body carries on many important functions or activities at the same time. All of these activities require cellular energy production. The memory, immune system, and even the DNA repair system are dependent on the proper production of cellular energy. This chapter will cover the benefits of NADH in these key areas.

Q. How does NADH help my body?

A. NADH has energy stored in its chemical structure. When it is absorbed and taken up by the body cells, NADH produces energy. NADH can be compared to a turbine in an electric power plant. Water at a higher level has more energy than water at a lower level. If you insert a turbine (wheel) in this waterfall, you can produce electrical energy. Hence, the more NADH a cell has available, the more energy can be produced. The amount of NADH a cell contains depends on the amount of energy the cell requires. Heart muscle cells have the highest NADH content because the heart is the organ that needs the most energy in the body. Cells in the brain and muscles contain 60 percent of the NADH content of those in the heart.

Q. Does NADH enhance the immune system?

A. Yes, it does. NADH is directly involved in the cellular immune defense system. Special white blood cells, called macrophages, are responsible for direct elimination of foreign bodies such as bacteria, viruses, and molds. They literally capture these foreign bodies and then degrade and eliminate them. During this process, a markedly increased metabolic activity including oxygen consumption takes place. Most of the oxygen is converted to superoxide and hydrogen peroxide, which are able to destroy viruses or bacteria. This phenomenon is known as "metabolic burst" and appears to be the first and most critical step leading to the destruction of the foreign invader. Large amounts of NADH are required for this process. Hence, the more NADH your body has available, the more protection your immune system can provide.

Q. How does NADH protect human cells within the body?

A. NADH empowers the body's natural repair mechanisms within cells. To explain in more detail, we are increasingly exposed to all kinds of harmful agents, toxins, chemicals, radiation, UV-light, ozone, and free radicals. All of these factors can damage the cell membrane or mitochondria where energy is both produced and stored. (Mitochondria are the energy-producing parts of cells.) These harmful agents can also damage the genetic material in all cells, which resides in the deoxyribonucleic acid (DNA). Replication of altered, defective DNA causes changed features in newly formed cells. The greater the DNA damage, the more extensive are the alterations in the cells and tissues. This is regarded as the biochemical cause of a number of chronic diseases such as cancer, rheumatoid arthritis, arteriosclerosis, and immunodeficiencies.

Fortunately, human cells have developed a system capable of repairing alterations of genetic material. This system is simply called the DNA repair system, which requires NADH to gain full functionality. Actually, at the innermost area of a cell (called the nucleus), there is only one known biological compound that can activate the nucleus DNA repair system: that compound is NADH. Therefore, the more NADH we have in our bodies, the better the DNA repair system functions, and the better we will be protected from developing degenerative diseases.

Q. Is NADH an antioxidant?

A. Yes, NADH actually is the body's most powerful antioxidant, and it can regenerate other important antioxidants to protect the body from damaging free-radical attack. NADH transfers the H (hydrogen) to oxidized (or damaged) glutathione to restore normal glutathione, one of the most important antioxidants produced in the body.

A similar situation exists for NADH (coenzyme 1) and vitamin-like coenzyme Q_{10} (CoQ_{10}). When CoQ_{10} is taken as a nutritional supplement, it is actually in an oxidized form and is therefore not an antioxidant. In the body, CoQ_{10} must be modified by NADH to become an effective antioxidant and also an energy-producing compound. Without the reductive (or transforming) ability of NADH, CoQ_{10} is useless to the body.

This ability of NADH to restore many other compounds into active, effective antioxidants is continuously being repeated in the body. For example, NADH restores used-up glutathione to its effective antioxidant form. This type of glutathione in turn can restore vitamin C back to its active state. Vitamin C in turn can regenerate used-up vitamin E back to active vitamin E. It is vital that the body have a sufficient supply of antioxidants such as NADH to eliminate dangerous free radicals, and it only takes a few milligrams (molecules) of NADH to have a profound influence on the body's antioxidant defense system against disease-causing free radicals.

Q. What type of damage can free radicals cause?

A. Free radicals are extremely reactive molecules that interact with many compounds in our cells, in particular with lipid-containing structures such as the cell membrane. For example, free radicals react with lipids surrounding the cell membrane, thereby violating the integrity of the cell wall, causing leakage and release of essential cellular components, which usually results in cell death. Free radicals have been shown to be involved in the development of cancer, coronary disease, atherosclerosis, diabetes, neurodegenerative disorders such as Parkinson's and Alzheimer's diseases, and other autoimmune diseases. Because NADH is an antioxidant by itself and a regenerator of other antioxidants, it's both a direct and indirect protector of human health.

Q. Can NADH enhance a person's memory?

A. Yes, it can. Memory is not a single function; rather, it's composed of a system of multiple processes. Memory can be defined as the storage of information, signals, and stimuli received by our five senses and the retrieval of this stored information. The major prerequisite for memory is cognition. Cognition is the process of receiving signals from outside the body. This is triggered by a chemical reaction in the cells of the central nervous system, and certain molecules induce information from one form to the other. These neurotransmitters are responsible for vegetative as well as cognitive performance. The best known neurotransmitters are adrenaline, its precursor noradrenaline, dopamine, and serotonin. With an increase in the production of these neurotransmitters, cognitive performance will improve. Several studies have shown that dopamine and adrenaline production are naturally increased by NADH. Therefore, NADH can effectively enhance memory.

Q. Are there more ways NADH can help?

A. Certainly. NADH provides several other health benefits. First, it protects the liver from alcohol damage. NADH is actually the cofactor (activator) of the enzyme that degrades alcohol (alcohol dehydrogenase). This means that the more NADH you have in your liver, the faster alcohol is eliminated. Additionally, NADH may improve the efficiency of liver enzyme functions, resulting in faster oxidation, shortened exposure, and reduced overall liver damage.

NADH also prevents the alcohol-induced inhibition of the sex hormone testosterone. Under the influence of alcohol, the production of the sex hormone testosterone is blocked. In other words, the more alcohol you consume, the lower your sex drive becomes. In the presence of NADH, this alcohol-induced inhibition of testosterone production is diminished or absent.

NADH lowers cholesterol levels and blood pressure. In a double-blind animal trial utilizing spontaneously hypertensive rats, NADH lowered cholesterol levels within eight weeks and reduced blood pressure within eleven weeks. These preliminary animal studies suggest that NADH has potential for lowering blood pressure and cholesterol levels in humans.

NADH inhibits dopamine auto-oxidation. The neurotransmitter dopamine is spontaneously oxidized in our bodies, in particular in the brain; this is called auto-oxidation. This process is found to be significantly higher in older individuals. Since NADH can inhibit the auto-oxidation of dopamine, it represents a useful tool in reducing or preventing damage to certain areas of the brain. Therefore, NADH may help retard cell death and tissue degeneration as we age.

4.

NADH for
Specific Conditions
and More

In just a few years, numerous studies and clinical trials have been conducted on NADH with impressive results. These studies, published in medical journals, have shown NADH's effectiveness or potential in treating a number of hard-to-treat conditions, including Parkinson's disease, chronic fatigue syndrome (CFS), Alzheimer's disease, and depression. This chapter will give you all the details on these conditions, how NADH has been found to help them, as well as how NADH can help healthy people and athletes.

Q. When was NADH first used therapeutically?

A. NADH was discovered more than ninety years ago, but it was not used therapeutically until 1985. That was when Dr. Walther Birkmayer and I began using NADH intravenously to treat patients with Parkinson's disease. The effect we saw from this treatment was phenomenal: patients who previously were unable to get up from their chairs could do so within an hour or two following intravenous infusion of NADH. The amazing effects we witnessed spurred us on to develop a stabilized, absorbable, oral tablet form of NADH, so that future patients and healthy people could have an effective form of NADH that they could use therapeutically and more conveniently.

Q. How does NADH help Parkinson's disease?

A. NADH has been found to dramatically help

the symptoms of Parkinson's disease, a progressive neurological disorder that affects about one million people in the United States, most of who are over the age of fifty. About fifty thousand new cases are reported each year. The age-specific incidence peaks at about age seventy and then declines. Men and women are equally affected, but African-Americans and Asians are less likely than whites to develop the disease.

The symptoms of Parkinson's disease are caused by a deficit in one of the most important messenger substances of the central nervous system, dopamine. This neurotransmitter is responsible for muscle tone and strength, upright position, libido, and emotional drive. This dopamine deficiency is reflected by the three major symptoms of Parkinson's disease: akinesia (inability to move), rigidity (stiffness), and tremors (shaking). These symptoms should not be ignored, as there is a reasonable and efficient treatment for Parkinson's disease, and life expectancy can be normal if the appropriate treatment is given.

It has been shown in a number of studies that NADH is able to stimulate the production of dopamine naturally. In an open-label clinical trial, 885 Parkinsonian patients were treated with the only stabilized, absorbable, oral form of NADH. After two weeks of treatment, a significant number of patients improved their mobility, particularly in the areas of walking, pushing, posture, speech, and mimics.

Q. Does NADH improve chronic fatigue syndrome?

A. Yes, NADH has been tested following strict Food and Drug Administration (FDA) and pharmaceutical testing guidelines, utilizing a double-blind, placebo-controlled, cross-over study that was performed at Georgetown University Medical Center in Washington, D.C. (A double-blind, placebo-controlled, crossover study means that neither the researchers nor the patients know who was taking NADH and who was taking the placebo; it is considered the gold standard of medical research.) The actual clinical findings, published in February 1999 in the *Annals of Allergy, Asthma and Immunology*, confirmed that

NADH is four times more effective than a placebo in relieving the symptoms of chronic fatigue syndrome.

Q. What exactly is chronic fatigue syndrome?

A. The name "chronic fatigue syndrome" was coined in 1988 by a group of scientists. Abbreviated CFS, the condition is also known as "chronic fatigue and immune dysfunction syndrome" (CFIDS) and "myalgic encephalomyelitis" (ME). It is a disorder of unknown etiology with a reported prevalence of up to three per every thousand people. An estimated 1 million Americans have the condition.

The syndrome is characterized by profound debilitating fatigue lasting at least six months, which often begins after a viral infection and which does not meet the criteria for other medical or psychiatric disorders. According to the Centers for Disease Control in Atlanta, Georgia, unexplained, debilitating fatigue of at least six months in duration must be present for a diagnosis of CFS, along with four or more of the following symptoms: impairment in short-term memory or concentration; muscle aches; sore throat; headache of a new type, pattern, or severity; prolonged exhaustion after exercising; joint pain; sleep disturbances or unrefreshing sleep; and swelling and tenderness of lymph nodes.

Q. Who is most likely to suffer from CFS?

A. Study data from the Centers for Disease Control (CDC) reported that historically over 90 percent of CFS sufferers are Caucasian and 85 percent are female. A new study published in the *Archives of Internal Medicine*, October 1999, found that CFS is a more common health condition than previously reported, especially for women across all ethnic groups. Further data suggests that approximately 75 percent of people with CFS have allergies while only 10 to 20 percent of the general population have allergies.

Q. Why would NADH be helpful for CFS?

A. All CFS sufferers complain about an overall lack of energy. As you'll recall, the body stores energy in the form of ATP. It has been demonstrated that CFS patients exhibit an ATP deficiency, particularly after even a low level of physical exercise. Therefore, a possible cause of chronic fatigue syndrome is a depletion of the cellular energy-storing molecule, ATP. An ATP deficiency is accompanied by severe fatigue, muscle weakness, and muscle pain—common symptoms of CFS. Rest and sleep offer no relief as minor exertions result in a continued debilitating tiredness. NADH can replenish the depleted cellular stores of ATP, thus improving the fatigue and cognitive dysfunction. Based on these observations, a double-blind, placebo-controlled, crossover study was launched at Georgetown University Medical Center using 10 mg of NADH. Since NADH increases ATP in cells, CFS patients in the study did benefit significantly from NADH treatment.

Q. What were the specific results of the study involving NADH and CFS?

A. Overall, the key finding in the study is that over 31 percent of the patients responded favorably to NADH after only four weeks of treatment by experiencing significant improvements in their symptoms. This results in NADH actually being four times more effective than a placebo. Additionally, in the longer-term open-label phase of the study, 72 percent of the patients continued to report an improvement of their symptoms after six months of taking 10 mg NADH daily. After approximately a year and a half of taking NADH, up to 81 percent of the patients continue to benefit from NADH.

"The four-fold increase in improvement in the NADH group is significant," explained Dr. Joseph Bellanti, the principal medical investigator of the Georgetown study. NADH is not a cure-all, but it can significantly relieve fatigue and improve concentration—two symptoms that seriously impair CFS patients' quality of life. "In conclusion, these findings suggest that long-term NADH therapy can lead to continued improvements, particularly in energy and mental/cognitive function."

Q. Is there anything else that's important to know about the Georgetown study?

A. The study was performed at the Georgetown University Medical Center only after an investigative new drug application was approved by the FDA. Based on this approval, the institutional review board of Georgetown University Medical Center gave approval for the study. A total of twenty-six eligible patients who fulfilled the Centers for Disease Control and Prevention criteria for CFS completed the study. Medical history, physical examination, laboratory studies, and questionnaires were obtained at baseline, four, eight, and twelve weeks. Subjects were randomly assigned to receive either 10 mg of NADH or a placebo for a four-week period followed by a four-week-washout period during which the subjects neither received NADH nor placebo. Subjects were then crossed over to the alternative regimen for a final four-week period in which the group receiving NADH in the first period received a placebo and the placebo group then received NADH. Therefore, neither the patients nor the administrators of the study knew, during the trial or evaluation, who was receiving which tablet.

Q. Is NADH's benefit for CFS really that important for society?

A. Absolutely. CFS is a very common health condition, especially among women across ethnic groups, and the costs to society are significant. Additional data from the recent study published in the *Archives of Internal Medicine* found that the incidence of CFS is at least twice as high as previously reported: It is estimated to affect about 836,000 people in the United States. Comparing the prevalence of CFS with other diseases in women, CFS emerges as a serious women's health concern, affecting 522 women per 100,000, as compared to breast cancer (26 per 100,000), lung cancer (33 per 100,000), and diabetes (900 per 100,000). The study also found that contrary to popular belief, elevated rates of CFS in Latinos and African Americans compared with the rates of CFS in whites.

CFS is also recognized by the National Institute of Health (NIH), Centers for Disease Control (CDC), Food and Drug Administration (FDA), and the Social Security Administration (SSA) as a serious, often disabling, illness. The SSA recently issued new guidelines for determining disability benefits for people with CFS. The estimated annual cost to the community for each person with chronic fatigue syndrome is $9,436. Nationwide, the community cost of CFS is staggering—almost $8 billion a year.

NADH has been proven to help improve energy levels in patients with this devastating condition. This means that the benefits of NADH treatment to individuals with CFS as well as to society as a whole could be enormous.

Q. Do any factors affect the amount of NADH CFS patients should take?

A. Large or overweight people may need higher dosages of NADH for the best effects. In a number of overweight CFS patient cases, researchers have found that 30 mg of NADH (six 5 mg tablets per day) leads to an improvement of CFS symptoms in four to six weeks. However, if some of these patients reduce the daily dosage to 10 mg, symptoms of CFS reappear.

Based on my experience with CFS patients, I recommend taking 10 mg of NADH (two 5 mg tablets) on a daily basis, in the morning and always on an empty stomach, with at least a half glass of water. If patients do not experience an improvement after four weeks of continuous usage, they should increase their dose to a third tablet either in the morning or early afternoon. They may also increase the daily dosage even further to four or five tablets, depending on their body size and weight and the severity of their symptoms. In other words, the optimum effective dosage of NADH varies according to each individual's own unique biochemistry and body makeup. Trial and error may be needed to find the best dosage for you.

Q. Were any side effects from NADH reported in the CFS study?

A. No. As an FDA-approved clinical trial, the Georgetown University Medical Center CFS study required careful documentation of any side effects or adverse reactions, but none were observed by the doctors or reported by patients. Side effects also were not reported in other studies—one involving 880 Parkinsonian patients who were treated with 10 to 25 mg of NADH orally or parentally for at least six months, and another involving 205 patients with depression.

Q. Is there a simple test to identify if I have CFS?

A. There may soon be. Another exciting result of the Georgetown University Medical Center

CFS Study was that medical researchers discovered a simple-to-test-for urinary predictive marker that may help doctors diagnose CFS in the future.

"One of the most frustrating aspects of the syndrome is that it is difficult to definitively diagnose," said Joseph A. Bellanti, MD, the chief investigator for the Georgetown study. "Findings from this study may now allow doctors to more quickly identify and treat CFS suffers."

The predictive marker is a neurotransmitter serotonin metabolite, called urinary 5-HIAA. The study tested urinary concentrations of twenty CFS patients and found that 75 percent of the subjects showed elevated levels of 5-HIAA. In seven of the ten NADH-treated subjects, the 5-HIAA levels returned to the normal range. In seven of the ten placebo-treated subjects, the 5-HIAA levels remained elevated or continued to increase.

The results of this preliminary study suggest that the measurement of urinary 5-HIAA may not only serve as a useful, simple-to-test-for predictive marker of the syndrome's activity in CFS patients, but may also provide an objective measure of the improvement following therapy with NADH. Additionally, testing of urinary 5-HIAA serves as a measure of improvement in neurocognitive dysfunction such as depression in CFS patients following therapeutic treatment with NADH.

Q. Could you give me an example of someone with CFS who has benefited from NADH?

A. There are many examples I could give you. The following is one case study provided by Dr. Ian Hyams, the assistant clinical director of the National ME Center at Harold's Wood Hospital in Romford, in the United Kindgom.

Diana Cannard, 61, of Stamford, Lincolnshire, was enjoying an active retirement, especially on the golf course, when she developed CFS following the second of two sinus operations in 1996. "The day before the operations, I was playing golf; the day after, I couldn't walk without excruciating pain in my leg muscles," explains Cannard. "Since then, I have suffered from a range of symptoms, including sleep disturbances, poor concentration, and severe muscle pain on walking and standing, and, if I overexert myself, a debiliting fatigue occurs. I experienced such difficulty concentrating that I couldn't absorb any new information, and I became very tired from simply talking or listening. All I could do socially was dine out with my husband—just a fraction of the range of social activities that I had enjoyed before. Whereas before I would walk around an eighteen-hole golf course wheeling a cart, now I can only walk twenty yards on a good day. I need a wheelchair outside the house though I can manage indoors, but I can only stand for about thirty seconds at a time."

Like many CFS patients, Cannard had tried a wide range of treatments for her condition. She gained some relief from the dreams and sleep disturbances that characterize her condition by taking a sleeping tablet and a low dose antidepressant. She also used a health point machine that stimulated acupressure points on the head and helped her relax and fall asleep more easily. She also saw a faith healer and began taking a daily cocktail of vitamins and minerals and following a strict diet to control *Candida albicans* (recurrent yeast infections).

Taking NADH has been the therapy that has been most beneficial for Cannard, though. "I have been taking 5 mg of NADH daily for two months. Just twenty-four hours after taking the first tablet, I woke up buzzing with energy and my enthusiasm returned," she says. "I have taken up my hobbies again, such as making toys. I can read, watch television, and even concentrate on serious documentaries and news programs. I am also much more sociable because talking and listening is a pleasure once again instead of being exhausting. NADH has returned my brain function to normal!"

Q. What kind of success with NADH supplementation are doctors seeing with CFS patients?

A. Perhaps Dr. Hyams, who has been using NADH to treat CFS patients for about one year, answers this question best. "Many patients have started on NADH as part of their treatment protocol and I have seen exciting results," Hyams says. "I hope this will be very good news for a large proportion of CFS sufferers. What excites me most of all is that NADH is a proven alternative for CFS patients to consider, particularly those patients who are sensitive to medication."

Q. Does NADH help with depression?

A. Yes, NADH improves the symptoms of depression, such as lack of enterprise, enjoyment, interest, concentration, reduced work capacity, loss of libido, and anxiety. Depression is an illness that causes a disturbance in an individual's emotions and feelings, referred to as mood. At any given time, approximately 5 percent of the population of the United States suffers from major depression. It affects people of all ages and ethnic groups. For unknown reasons, women are almost twice as likely as men to suffer from depression. The lifetime prevalence of major depression is about 20 to 26 percent for women and 8 to 12 percent for men. Those who have had an episode of depression have better than a 50 percent chance of the depression recurring sometime in their lives. It can occur at any age; however, the average age of onset is about forty years old. Although many people experience their first episode of depression in their late teens or early adulthood, the incidence of depression increases with age. The elderly are at a high risk of developing depression as they face multiple health problems or the loss of loved ones.

Q. How do I know if I have depression and can benefit from NADH?

A. Medical practitioners consider nine classic symptoms when diagnosing depression. A patient must have five or more of the following symptoms during the same two-week period: depressed mood for most of the day; disturbed appetite or change in weight; disturbed sleep; psychomotor retardation or agitation; loss of interest in previously pleasurable activities; fatigue or loss of energy; feelings of worthlessness or excessive and/or inappropriate guilt; difficulty concenrating or thinking clearly; and morbid or suicidal thoughts or actions. At least one of the five symptoms must be either a depressed mood or loss of interest or pleasure.

The absolute causes of depression are not totally identified, but imbalances in neurotransmitters (chemicals in the nervous system) such as dopamine, norepinephrine, and serotonin play a key role in depression. Because NADH is known to stimulate the natural production of these neurotransmitters, an initial pilot study consisting of 205 patients suffering from depression was conducted. The patients were given 10 mg of NADH on a daily basis for 5 to 310 days. Impressively, 93 percent of the depressed patients exhibited a beneficial clinical effect.

If you have depression—especially if you have suicidal thoughts—it's important that you work with a mental health therapist who knows your individual case and history. Given the positive results demonstrated with NADH for depression, NADH may very well help you with depression, but be sure to discuss this with your doctor.

Q. Will NADH help with dementia and Alzheimer's disease?

A. Yes, NADH has been shown to improve cognitive impairment. In an FDA-approved, double-blind, placebo-controlled study performed at Georgetown University Medical Center, it was found that patients with dementia of the type found in Alzheimer's disease showed a statistically significant improvement after six months of treatment using 10 mg dosage (two 5 mg NADH tablets) daily. Patients treated with NADH showed no evidence of progressive cognitive decline during the period of treatment and demonstrated significant improvement on measures of memory, verbal fluency, and visual-perceptual problem solving. These results support the use of NADH as part of the Alzheimer's disease treatment program. The results may reflect improving energy metabolism in damaged but still viable brain cells.

Based on these results, NADH may hold promise for treating elderly people who suffer from Alzheimer's disease. Approximately 4 to 5 million Americans—5 to 11 percent of Americans over the age of 65 and approximately 50 percent of the population over the age of 85—have been diagnosed with Alzheimer's. This disease causes such progressive loss of function that more than 50 percent of these people require institutional care that is estimated to cost society billions of dollars. If future studies confirm that NADH can hold off mental decline in the dementia seen in Alzheimer's, this could improve the quality of life of Alzheimer's patients and of society as a whole.

Q. Is NADH helpful for athletes?

A. Given that athletes use more energy than non-athletes, it makes sense that a substance like NADH, which improves energy production, might boost athletes' energy levels and result in improved performance. In an initial pilot study of four highly trained elite-class athletes, each was given NADH as a supplement to enhance performance of both short-term and prolonged exercise at maximal intensity. The study demonstrated that all the athletes improved both their short-term and long-duration performance levels up to 13 percent after only two months of supplementing with 10 mg of NADH (two 5 mg tablets) per day. Other studies have also shown that cyclists increased their oxygen capacity and improved their reaction times after only one month of 5 mg of NADH per day.

Normal weekend-type athletes can customize the amount of NADH they take daily by tailoring dosage levels to suit their overall health or training needs. When taking NADH for athletic activities or training, make certain that you take NADH (minimum 5 mg daily) for at least one month prior to the event; this will allow for optimum energy effectiveness at the cellular level. Longer-term usage should result in improved oxygen capacity, increased reaction time, and greater mental acuity and alertness.

Q. Can healthy people benefit by taking NADH?

A. Most certainly. Healthy people can and do

benefit from taking NADH. The body makes small amounts of NADH, but just about everybody can benefit from increased or more efficient energy production. Younger, healthy individuals may supplement their intake with the lowest dosage—2.5 mg—which seems to fulfill the body's need for NADH. However, as people get older, the body's ability to make NADH declines, and supplementation at 5 mg and higher on a daily basis can prove to be beneficial.

To date, more than 75 percent of consumers taking NADH for one to three months report an increase in physical and mental energy. Normal healthy individuals will also benefit from the protection against potential cell damaging agents such as toxins, pollutants, food additives, radiation, and free radicals that NADH provides.

Q. Can NADH be considered an anti-aging nutrient?

A. Yes, NADH has significant anti-aging potential. Aging is a highly complex biological process associated with a progressive decline in the performance of many organs in the body. As we age, the NADH and energy levels in our cells decrease. In other words, aging is loss of energy. When cellular energy declines below a certain threshold, cells in our bodies begin to slowly deteriorate and tissue begins to degenerate. This energy loss can also signal the beginning of more serious illnesses later in life. As I have noted in previous chapters, there is growing evidence that a lack of cellular energy may accelerate the aging process, ultimately resulting in degenerative diseases, such as Alzheimer's, cancer, and many others. Conversely, if the cell is producing adequate energy, it can continue to perform all of its processes more efficiently. The more NADH a cell has available, the more energy it will produce and the longer it will continue to properly function. NADH's further anti-aging potential is derived from the fact that NADH is one of the strongest, most powerful biological antioxidants and, therefore, helps protect cells from damaging agents and free radicals that can age the body.

5.

How and When to Take NADH

NADH is essential for adequate energy, and supplementation can improve energy levels. Knowing exactly what type of NADH to take and how and when to take it, though, is vital information you must know so that you can get the best results possible. In this chapter, you'll learn all about NADH supplementation—the best type, its safety, and how best to take NADH to achieve effective results.

Q. What's the best NADH to buy?

A. There is only one stabilized, absorbable form available that increases NADH levels in cells.

ENADA is the only brand of NADH currently available that is stabilized and is actually protected by several worldwide patents. Competitors continue to try to bypass these patents and introduce NADH products. However, all these products are non-stabilized forms of NADH. When subjected to independent laboratory analysis and validation, the majority of these products do not contain any NADH. The result of the absence of NADH in these products hurts consumers and leaves the impression that NADH is ineffective. Remember, if an NADH product isn't stabilized, you're wasting your money.

Q. How safe is NADH?

A. NADH is a very safe biological compound. Remember, NADH occurs in high concentration in many tissues and organs, particularly in the heart, brain, and muscles. All living cells must have NADH or the cell will deteriorate and not function. Tests have shown that over seven thousand times the daily recommended dosage can be tolerated with virtually no significant side effects. On the basis of this value, NADH can be regarded as one of the safest biological substances.

Q. Is there data on safe dosage levels for NADH?

A. Yes. To begin clinical trials, the FDA requires that safety data test results be presented for approval before any human trials can be scheduled. Toxicology safety studies on NADH were performed, and they found that the maximum tolerated dosage of NADH is 500 mg per kg of body weight per day. The dosage applied to clinically studied patients was 10 mg per patient per day; this is regarded as a totally safe and acceptable therapeutic dosage. Based on the safety data, the maximum tolerated human dosage is more than 3,500 times higher than the 10 mg dosage given to the CFS patients. It should be noted that the majority of the patients in my clinical practice have been taking between 10 and 30 mg of NADH on a daily basis for over four years without any adverse reactions. In other words, NADH is an extremely safe substance.

Q. Are there any side effects from taking NADH?

A. Since the introduction of NADH in the early 1990s, the safety of NADH continues to be supported by several types of clinical data. First, the FDA approved two human clinical trials and any side effects found in these trials were required to be fully documented. The results of these trials were that not a single side effect was reported. In addition, more than three thousand patients have received stabilized NADH for treatment of therapeutic conditions since the late 1980s. No side effects have been observed in these patients. It's also important to know that hundreds of thousands of consumers have taken NADH since it was made available in health food stores and pharmacies in the United States more than four years ago, and consumers have reported no significant side effects.

Q. Can I take NADH with medication?

A. Yes, you can take NADH with medication, including the most common antihypertensive, antidepressive, and antihistaminic drugs. In one of the FDA-approved clinical trials, many patients were on antihypertensive and/or antidepressive and/or antihistaminic drugs. No interference was observed with these medications. However, be sure to check with your health care professional for his or her advice.

Q. When is the best time to take NADH?

A. The best time to take NADH is first thing in the morning on an empty stomach, 30 minutes before any food, drugs, or other supplements, with a glass of water. The NADH tablets are enteric coated and are designed to bypass the stomach and "float" with water into the intestine where absorption takes place. If you need additional energy for the late afternoon or evening, you can also take an additional NADH tablet either thirty minutes before lunch or about two hours after lunch, and again, at least thirty minutes before a late afternoon snack or an early dinner. It is important that NADH is taken on an empty stomach so it can easily "flush" or move into the intestines where it is absorbed.

Q. How soon should I expect to see results with NADH?

A. The answer to this question varies according to the individual. Each of us has a very unique biochemistry: Our bodies absorb food and nutrients differently, and our metabolisms often differ in other dramatic ways.

On average, optimal effectiveness is shown in four weeks of continuous usage. However, many healthy individuals report an improvement in energy levels within five to ten days. NADH must enter the billions of cell structures for energy production to begin, so first-time users may need to be patient before seeing beneficial results.

Q. How long should I take NADH?

A. For normal healthy people who are taking NADH for increased daily energy and mental clarity, optimal effectiveness is achieved within one month of continuous usage. One month, therefore, is the minimum time period to take the product. After one month of continuous usage, normal healthy individuals who supplement with NADH for energy can try using it on an every-other-day basis. However, it is best to take NADH daily.

Research suggests that NADH can be taken safely for long periods of time. Many people have been taking NADH for several years with no side effects reported. The body is in a continuous state of refueling itself with cellular energy and NADH is a very efficient cellular energizer. So, the more NADH the body has available, the more the body will use to produce more energy. If you are taking NADH therapeutically, continuous daily usage is recommended. However, it is always best to check with your health care provider to help monitor long-term usage of any supplement.

6.

NADH
Survey Results

As you now know, NADH has been sold in the United States as a dietary supplement since 1995. To find out what people experience after using the product for at least one month, a research survey was conducted among 5,000 NADH users. This chapter will cover the real-life uses and benefits of NADH based on results from that survey.

Q. What are the main reasons people take NADH?

A. More than 51 percent of users who take NADH do so for energy enhancement. They are truly tired of being tired. Twenty percent are using NADH for chronic fatigue, a debilitating lack of energy; 13 percent take NADH for disease conditions such as Parkinson's disease, fibromyalgia (severe muscle pain and tenderness), and Alzheimer's disease; and another 16 percent take NADH for a variety of other medical or health-related reasons.

Q. What percentage of people experience good results with NADH after just one month?

A. An overwhelming 84 percent of people surveyed reported "some to substantial" improvement for what they are taking NADH for—primarily, increased energy—after only one month of taking NADH. Lack of energy is a nearly universal complaint in doctors' offices, so this data is very encouraging: NADH supplementation may help improve the energy levels and, therefore, the quality of life of many people.

Q. What is the most common dosage taken by users of NADH?

A. Slightly more than 74 percent of people who take NADH take it daily, while 16 percent are taking it twice a day and 7 percent are taking it less than daily. However, 3 percent of those who supplement with NADH are using more than two tablets daily. Again, usage is dependent on whether consumers are taking NADH for overall energy or for therapeutic reasons.

Q. Can you share any case summaries of consumer experiences with NADH?

A. I'll describe four case studies. The first one concerns Stephanie W., a twenty-four-year-old waitress who was diagnosed with chronic fatigue syndrome at the age of sixteen. She experienced symptoms of the illness for years, and by the time she arrived at college in Connecticut, the overall tiredness and lethargy was severe. While she was in college, her mother, who owns a health food store, found out about the Georgetown University study on NADH and convinced Stephanie to begin taking the product. After eight weeks, she found she was not as tired, much more alert, and better able to concentrate. Previously, Stephanie had experienced symptoms of blurred vision and muscle joint pain and those went away after two months. At present, Stephanie currently takes 15 mg of NADH on a daily basis.

Devora B., who was diagnosed with CFS five years ago, is another case study. Formerly a TV producer, Devora started to lose the energy that was required for her fast-paced job. She decided to adopt a child and stop working, even though she knew that raising a child also requires a certain amount of stamina. Eventually she was diagnosed with CFS, and she began learning about supplements. Although she couldn't figure out what was wrong with her, she decided to network with other CFS sufferers to explore the baffling nature of this condition. Four months ago, she learned about NADH and the study at Georgetown University. She started taking 10 mg NADH daily. Within a week, she noticed an improvement in the way she felt. Then, all of a sudden, she had so much more energy to take care of her adopted child—something she is truly grateful for.

Another encouraging case history involves Cynthia M., who was feeling "quite awful," as she described, for over six weeks. Cynthia's doctor said she might have either fibromyalgia or CFS, conditions that are believed to be incurable, and just thinking about being stricken with such a lack of energy forever was awful. Cynthia went to see an endocrinologist, an arthritis specialist, and a gynecologist, hoping for a second opinion, but ended up feeling like she had wasted her time. She listened to her doctor and rested, exercised, and ate well, adding vitamins to her diet. Eventually she felt better, but a few weeks later, the "icky feelings" returned.

One day, Cynthia was reading through a newspaper when she came across a news clip on the Georgetown study of NADH. The study recommended that if you plan to take more than 5 mg of NADH, you should contact your doctor, so Cynthia contacted hers right away. She went to a health food store and began to add NADH to her other supplements. Just one week later, Cynthia exclaimed, "I felt 100 percent better!"

Finally, consider the story of Gerry Y., who lives at and works on a farm and horse ranch with her husband in Ohio. Gerry had always been somewhat of a "health nut" who focused on natural remedies, but six years ago, to her dismay, she was diagnosed with chronic leukemia. Gerry was adamantly opposed to taking any drugs if it were possible to treat her condition naturally. So, Gerry began to do some research, determined to beat the constant fatigue and weakness present with her condition with a natural remedy.

One day, Gerry saw NADH on the counter of a local pharmacy and decided to try it. Two weeks later, Gerry noticed a definite improvement. Before taking NADH, she would have to lie down two to three times a day; now she spends twelve to fourteen hours on her horse farm riding and cleaning out stalls! Gerry usually takes 5 mg NADH, but if she knows that she's got a tough day ahead of her, she'll take 10 mg. Gerry says that she does not have to lie down and take naps anymore. She rides better and her riding instructor has noticed the improvement and is very impressed. She says her mind is so much sharper and she looks better, and people never believe she has leukemia.

Consider these case studies: NADH has helped improve the energy level of people from all walks of life; it just might help you.

Conclusion

NADH is beneficial for every human being. Studies show that whether you are a highly conditioned athlete or a person suffering from chronic fatigue syndrome, Alzheimer's disease or other disease conditions, NADH may be helpful. The majority of us have normal health that falls somewhere between the health of these various groups, so NADH likely can benefit all of us.

This book answers and explains the many questions and important roles that NADH plays in our bodies. The most important of these, of course, is to increase cellular energy. NADH also enhances the immune system and protects the cells from damage by free radicals, chemical toxins, radiation and other damaging compounds. Published studies on NADH's ability to be a beneficial and powerful antioxidant have convinced me that NADH has remarkable health-protective benefits.

I have been taking 5 mg a day of NADH since its development in the early 1990s. Since then, I have never caught the flu or any other infectious disease, and my physical and mental energy levels have increased considerably. Considering the safety and impressive research behind NADH, I'm confident that this remarkable supplement can help a great many people in similar ways as it has done for me. Talk to your health care professional about including NADH into your daily supplements. Follow the dosage recommendation, and you will be surprised how NADH can help change your life for the better.

Glossary

Adenosine triphosphate (ATP). The primary energy currency of a cell derived from the metabolism of glucose, amino acids, fatty acids, and the reaction of oxygen with NADH.

Antidepressants. Pharmaceutical agents used to treat clinical depression.

Anti-inflammatory. Agents that reduce inflammation without directly antagonizing the agent that caused it.

Antioxidant. A substance that combines with free radicals, neutralizing them, and thus prevents the deterioration of DNA, RNA, lipids, and proteins.

Autoimmune disease. A disorder in which the body mounts a destructive immune response against its own tissue.

Bioavailability. The rate at which a nutrient is made available for action in the body.

Cell. The smallest organized unit of living structure in the body. There are trillions of cells making up the human body.

Cholesterol. The most abundant steroid in tissue. Used to make hormones in the body. The liver can manufacture cholesterol.

Chronic fatigue immune dysfunction syndrome (CFIDS). A synonym for chronic fatigue syndrome used by patients and physicians.

Coenzyme. A substance that enhances or is necessary for the action of an enzyme. They are generally a much smaller molecule than enzymes.

Depression. A neurotic or psychotic condition marked by an inability to concentrate, possible insomnia, and feeling of dejection and guilt.

Dopamine. A neurotransmitter responsible for a sense of well-being and for energizing the body. It stimulates strength, coordination, cognition, mood, sex drive, and growth hormone secretion.

Enzyme. Specialized proteins that act as catalysts for virtually all necessary chemical reactions that take place within the body.

Fibromyalgia. Also known as myofascial pain syndrome and fibromyositis. A group of common rheumatoid disorders characterized by achy pain, tenderness, and stiffness of muscles.

Free radical. A molecule that lacks an electron and aggressively seeks to replace it. Free radicals can cause cellular oxidation and inhibit normal functioning of cells and can lead to many diseases.

Metabolism. The chemical and physical processes continuously occurring in the body, involving the creation and breakdown of molecules.

Mitochondria. The chemical factories of cells, where energy is made. Often referred to as the outer layer of the cell structure.

Myalgic encephalomyelitis (ME). A synonym for chronic fatigue syndrome in common usage in the United Kingdom and Canada.

Neurotransmitters. Substances produced in neurons that promote or inhibit the conduction of nerve impulses, such as norepinephrine, dopamine, and serotonin.

Norepinephrine. A neurotransmitter responsible for alertness, concentration, and mental activity.

Oxidation. The process by which a compound reacts with oxygen and loses an electron.

Placebo. A dummy pill that contains no active ingredient such as a sugar pill.

Serotonin. A neurotransmitter important for sleep and emotional balance.

References

Birkmayer GD, Birkmayer W. "The coenzyme nicotinamide adenine dinucleotide (NADH) as biological antidepressive agent experience with 205 patients." *New Trends in Clinical Neuropharmacology* 1991; 5:75–86.

Birkmayer JGD. "Stable, ingestable and absorbable NADH and NADPH therapeutic compositions," United States Patent No. 5.332.727. 1994.

Birkmayer JGD, Birkmayer W. "Stimulation of the endogenous L-dopa biosynthesis—a new principle for the therapy of Parkinson's disease: the clinical effect of nicotinamide adenine dinucleotide (NADH) and nicotinamide adenine dinucleotidephosphate (NADPH)." *Acta Neurologica Scandinavica,* 1989; 126:183–187.

Birkmayer W, Birkmayer JGD, Vrecko C, Paletta B, Reschenhofer E, Ott E. "Nicotinamide adenine dinucleotide (NADH) as medication for Parkinson's disease. Experience with 415 patients." *New Trends in Clinical Neuropharmacology* 1990; 4(1): 7–24.

Birkmayer W, Rieder P. *Understanding the Neurotransmitters: Key to the Workings of the Brain.* Springer Verlag: Wien-New York, 1989.

Busheri N, Taylor J, Lieberman S, Mirdamadi-Zonosi N, Birkmayer G, Preuss HG. "Oral NADH affects blood pressure, lipid peroxidation and lipid profile in spontaneously hypertensive rats." *Journal of the American College of Nutrition.* 1997.

Hazleton Europe Report No. 1174/1-1050: Final Report, "Birmadil (NADH): Single intravenous administration toxicity study in the rat," for Labor Birkmayer & MEDINFO GesmbH, 1994.

Kuhn W, Müller Th, Winkel R, Danielczik S, Gerstner A, Häcker R, Mattern C, Przuntek H. "Parenteral application of NADH in Parkinson's disease: Clinical improvement partially due to stimulation of endogenous levodopa biosynthesis." *Journal of Neural Transmission.* 1996; 103: 1187–1193.

Leonard A. Jason, PhD; Judith A. Richman, PhD; Alfred W. Rademaker, PhD; Karen M. Jordan, PhD; Audrius V. Pilioplys, MD; Renee R. Taylor, PhD; William McCready, PhD; Cheng-Fang Huang, MS; Sigita Pilioplys, MD. "A Community-Based Study of chronic fatigue syndrome" *Archives of Internal Medicine.* 1999; 159: 2129–2137.

Suggested Reading

Birkmayer George, *NADH—The Energizing Coenzyme*. New Canaan, CT: Keats Publication, 1998.

Index